Table of Contents

Introduction

    The Importance of Essential Oils

Chapter One: The Production and Usage of Essential Oils

    Comparing Essential Oils Quality

    Purchasing and Storing your Essential Oils

    How to store essential oils to ensure longevity

    Do Essential oils have expiry dates?

    Basics of Essential oils storage

Chapter Two: Applying Essential Oils

    Methods of Application

    Internal use of Essential Oils

    Why you will need to take caution with essential oil

    Major Essential oils and associated side effects

    Blending Essential Oils

    Essential Oils Notes

    Carrier Oil

    Diffusers

    Types of Diffusers

    Benefits of using Diffusers

    Safety Measures with Essential Oils

Chapter Three: Basic Essential Oils You Will Need

    Lavender Oil

    Rosemary Oil

    Peppermint Oil

    Lemon Oil

    Chamomile Roman Oil

    Thyme Oil

Tea Tree Oil

Chapter Four: Essential Oils for Health Care

Liver Cleanse

Stomach Ache

Muscle Pain

Cuts, Burns and Bruises

Common Cold and Flu

Oral Health

Headaches

Heartburn

Palpitations

Whitlows

Anal Fissures

Black eyes

Bleeding

Boils

Blisters

Catarrh

Chapter Five: Essential Oils for Children

Essential Oils for Baby/Toddler Phase

Safety precautions for using essential oils on babies

Essential oils for babies between the ages of 4 months to 1-year-old

Essential oils for Children

Chapter Six: Essential oils for Skin Care

Essential oils for Face Masks

Facial steaming using essential oils

Facial Toner with Essential oils

Facial scrub with essential oils

Essential Oils used for Hair Care

Chapter Seven: Essential Oils for Home Use
        Common Essential Oils for Home Use
        Parts of the home and essential oils that suit them best
        The Bedroom
        The Living Room
        The Bathroom
Chapter Eight: Essential Oils for Emotional Wellbeing
        Essential Oils for Calmness
        Essential Oils to help with bereavement
        Essential Oils for Stress Control
        Essential Oils for Depression
Conclusion

Introduction

Mother Nature is vast and abundant, with numerous blessings for us humans dwelling here in her bowls (earth). One such thing that she has blessed us with is the beautiful gift of essential oils. Essential oils in the most basic form can be described as natural elements having sweet-smelling qualities that are flattering to the olfactory system of the body. Most of these have not only the quality of pleasant aroma but also anti-bacterial and anti-inflammatory qualities that make them very effective in dealing with infections. Some others also possess qualities capable of influencing human mood and emotional stability. They are known as essential oils because they contain the essence of a plant's fragrance.

The special scent and aroma that oozes from various herbs and spices and gives them their distinct taste and flavor are all from the essential oils contained inside of them. These oils can also be found in fruits, which helps to provide them with their unique tastes and aroma whenever they are squeezed, cut open, or peeled. One example that comes to mind is the distinct smell that fills the air whenever the orange peel is squeezed.

Aromatherapy, which is the study of essential oils and their aromatic qualities, has been in practice for years and centuries, leading to the production of perfumes, praying incenses, and cosmetics. Some of these are so powerful that they are employed in religious rituals, such as the frankincense used by the Roman Catholic during mass. The ancient people of India made use of aromatic herbs such as cinnamon, sandalwood, and ginger for therapeutic purposes. The Chinese employed aromatics to help out with the acupuncture process.

Further back in time, it has also been discovered that the Egyptians made use of perfumes and fine oils to 'gladden' the gods. Others, such as cedar and myrrh, were used in the embalming of dead Pharaohs.

All of these are clear pointers to the fact that essential oils were a pricey commodity in the ancient world.

Early merchants traded these aromatic oils because they were quite rare and sometimes difficult to produce. The aromatic oils played a significant role in the history of the Israelites and the ordination of the biblical Priests and Levis. Throughout their time in the wilderness, the Bible recorded that Yahweh gave Moses some special instructions concerning the usage of some essential oils in the production of the anointing oil, which they used in the consecration of the new Priests to set them apart for their spiritual work.

The critical history of the aromatic and essential oils boomed in the eastern world until Arabian merchants introduced the west to this wealth during their numerous trade sessions. The Greeks also got into the equation, learning lots of secrets about the preparation of these perfumes from Egyptians. The first recorded instance of turpentine distillation was carried out by a Greek known as Herodotus. Other notable names include Hippocrates, who cured some of his sick patients with concussions made from the mixture of these essential oils.

Over the years, the various uses and importance of different essential oils have been documented by Pharmacists who have carried out credible experiments. In our modern world, the perfumery industry has blown up to attract lots of innovative scientific and medical minds. The essential oils are some of the major components of pharmaceutic drugs used in the treatments of various ailments.

With the modernization of this industry, the core natural, herbal, and traditional methods of using essential oils for treatment lost its place. But in recent times, the benefits of raw essential oils and their usage has started regaining its place in the medical industry.

The Importance of Essential Oils

Some of the chemical components contained in our bodies are also contained in essential oils. Some of these are naturally occurring in the body, and they are known to help out in the daily functioning of the body's system. Most of them are produced during normal body metabolism. Some of these components are also produced as essential in plants. When into the human body, they help to augment the already available quantity of these components in the body.

Most of these essential oils produced by plants are hardly ever toxic to the human. However, you will need to seek professional advice regarding dosage while making use of these oils because they can create adverse reactions when misused. But looking on the bright side, most of these essential oils have found to have the ability to heal, to revive the human mood, and also keep off some predators. In this modern world, with all of the advancements that have made in the aromatherapy industry, more and more essential oils are being discovered that serve lots of important purposes.

Centuries of research have shown that most of these essential oils have antineuralgic, antirheumatic, and analgesic qualities. Essential oils can be applied or used in a variety of ways, such as by inhalation, ingestion, or external application on the body. The method used depends solely on the rate of absorption of the particular essential oil to be applied.

Aside from the health industry, essential oils are also actively used in the food packaging industry as preservatives. Their flavors are also quite important in the production of sweets and drinks. In the cosmetics industry, they are loved for their cell rejuvenating qualities.

In this book, we are going to exploring some of the most interesting and important uses of essential oils as they relate to your everyday life. Lots of people have no idea that having a basic knowledge of essentials oils and their applications can help you save some money when you decide to produce finished products with them. Some of them can even be grown in a small garden behind your house so that they can be easily plucked for usage.

Chapter One: The Production and Usage of Essential Oils

Essential oils are produced or extracted from plants using different methods. The principle of these extractions relies heavily on the fact that these essential oils are known to blend well when they are mixed with other oils or alcohols. Producers have discovered that some essential oils are best extracted with one method of extraction over others. It is the understanding of these essential oils and their best extraction methods that makes it easier to extract them. Some of the most popular extraction methods include:

Expression

This is one of the most common methods of extracting essential oils from plants. It basically involves the pressing of the plant's seeds until the oil oozes out. This method is that which is mostly used in the extraction of oils from citrus fruits such as oranges and lemons.

Using Solvents

This kind of extraction relies on the difference in boiling point between the essential oils and the solvents used in the extraction. In this method, the plant source is dissolved in the solvents and then boiled. The solvent will evaporate, leaving the essential oils in the container. A centrifuge is then used to separate the essentials oil from the solvent. Although this method works all the time, most essential oil producers detest the method believing that it affects the quality of the finished produced. The essential oils produced this way are usually referred to as absolutes.

The Steam Distillation Method
This method is probably the most popular method of essential oil extraction used by aromatherapists. In this process, the plant is placed in a still, and steam is passed through it to create concentrated vapor. While this happens, aromatic pockets are opened that help to release the essential oils into the steam. Precaution must be taken so that the steam isn't too hot enough to destroy the plant source. If not, the whole process goes to waste. The steam is then condensed until a mixture of water; then, the essential oil is gotten. The oil, being immiscible with water, floats at the top where it can easily be separated from the water.

Comparing Essential Oils Quality
If you are going to be using essential oils, then it is necessary that you know how to verify the quality of whatever oil you may intend to use for whatever purpose. The quality of essential oils varies, and this variation will have an effect on the results gotten when they are used. For a novice user, it can be quite hard to verify the quality of oils before they are used. These oils travel from far places in the world to meet you, the consumer. Some farmers, looking to make a quick profit over a short period, will put out low-quality products into the market. The question now is: How can you prevent yourself from falling prey to their antics. Here are some ways you can do just that.

Know the Latin name of your favorite essential Oils: While looking to purchase essential oils for your use, you will come across a lot of them that look and smell like the one you are trying to get, sometimes with similar general names. This is where your knowledge of their botanical names comes in. Read the label of the oils and check if the botanical names on the bottle are the same with what you are looking to get.

The Grading System: There is a grading system that exists for essential oils, and it varies from one manufacturer/producer to the next. The cost of any essential oil is mostly determined by its grade. This grading system is generally used to specify which of these oils is best for a particular use. It will be quite impossible for you to master the grades all at once, but as time goes on, you will get used to this grading system and understand how it works.

The Price Tag: some of the major distributors understand that most consumers are on the lookout for the best essential oils for the lowest prices. They have a kind of sweet-mouth that can help them convince buyers that a particular oil they sell is the best that can be found anywhere in the world for the price being offered. Don't fall prey to this.

One thing you should understand is that quality essential oils will always be expensive, considering the efforts required in extracting some of them. For example, it takes about 60 roses to produce a few drops of rose essential oil. It is only natural that it will be more expensive than other more abundant oils. Stay clear of producers who use the same price for quality across all oils.

Oil Integrity: The integrity of an essential oil refers to the percentage of purity of oil from its natural source. These oils are not produced in laboratories or with a mixture of other oils that smell almost like them. Whenever an essential oil is mixed with other pure essential oils to make them smell and look more qualitative, they instantly lose their integrity. Other times they are mixed with alcohol to improve their smell. Even with them, essential oil experts are always able to identify the presence of alcohol by merely sniffing a bottle.

As a beginner or a novice, you can carry out your test by placing a drop of the oil on a sheet of white paper. For oils with integrity, there will be no oily spot on the paper after the fragrance has evaporated after 24 hours. If there is a presence of oiliness after evaporation, it simply proves that the oil has no integrity.

Purchasing and Storing your Essential Oils
After verifying the integrity of both the oil and its supplier, you may want to keep them for future supplies. Most companies are known for their constant supply of quality, and some others are famed for adulteration. Of course, those known for quality will always charge more for their products, but the truth is that you will never regret making that purchase.

One of the most important things you can do before making a purchase is to do a background check on companies who sell these oils, especially if you are making your purchase off the internet. If all of the things contained in this book are going to help out in your application of essential oils, then the first thing you will need to get right is the purchase of quality oils. Adulterated packages will always produce low-quality products and leave you with regrets. One way to check for the quality of essential oil and the accountability of the company distributing it is by the quality of packaging. Essential oils are best packaged in dark-colored glass bottles to prevent evaporation. Only serious and genuine sellers know this and go through the stress of packaging their essential oils with the right quality. If you come across essential oils packaged in plastic bottles, then you should have it in the mind that it is most certainly fake. Take your money somewhere else.

How to store essential oils to ensure longevity

The storage process is one-factor people rarely consider when dealing with essential oils. How long your oils maintain their quality and beneficial properties depend largely on the method of storage, you adopt with them. When they are stored in the right way, most of them are capable of retaining their qualities for even up to a year. Some are capable of lasting as long as five years if they are stored in the right way.

Do Essential oils have expiry dates?

Essential oils can expire, lose their essence, and become unsafe for usage. Whenever essential oils are not stored properly, they become exposed to oxidation, which makes them lose their aroma and whatever beneficial qualities they once had. Essentials oils all have varying lengths before degradation begins. For some, they may need only months before they begin to lose their essence. For others, they even get stronger and more potent as they age and then begin to lose essence after a while. The duration before degradation and loss of essence begins wholly on the source plant of the oils, the method of extraction, and the initial integrity level.

Some ways you can tell that essential oil has lost its essence include loss of aroma, change in color, foggy look in a glassy container, and thick consistency.

Basics of Essential oils storage
The first thing you have to understand about essential oils if you are ever going to store them properly is that they hate the sunlight. Sunlight heat is capable of affecting their chemical composition, causing them to evaporate and cause faster degradation of the oil. For this reason, it is best to store essential oils in dark-colored glass bottles that will help to keep sunlight out.

Essential oils should never be stored in plastic bottles if you want to preserve them for longevity. One popular bottle color choice has been the dark amber glass bottle. You can find various shades of bottle colors that can help you achieve this. Find one that suits your style and go with it.

Also, don't keep the bottles in a place where sunlight might reach them, even if they are contained in dark-colored glass bottles. The bottle will heat up and still affect the oil quality as time goes on. Find a dark and cool spot in the house where the oxidation process will be reduced drastically. It is better to store essential oils in glass bottles than plastic bottles because they are very potent, and some are capable of reacting with the plastic bottles and dissolving them.

Another option is to cool them. The temperature reduction helps to reduce the oxidation process. Make some space in your refrigerator and store up the bottles. Don't allow them to get frozen. Remember that isn't the point of storage in the refrigerator; it is basically to keep them cool.

Remember to take the bottle off the fridge some hours before you use them, so they regain room temperature application.

The aromatherapy box is another option you can explore while trying to store your bottles of oil. It doesn't have to be something large and fanciful. Something portable and padded should be enough to get the job done. Before sending them back into the boxes, remember to tighten the lids so that the oils don't sip and waste.

Chapter Two: Applying Essential Oils

As we have noted earlier, there are many uses of essential oils, and you, as a first time user has to define your purpose of usage so that you can make the most of your oils. Find out that the oil you have purchased is perfect for the need to have to satisfy.

Another important point to note is if there are any side effects associated with the usage of essential oil. What are the precautions that should be taken before, during, and after use? You can either get this information from your doctor, supplier, or container. Also, stay observant during application so you can easily spot any adverse reaction and discontinue usage.

Methods of Application

There are three basic ways in which essential oils can be applied to the skin. They include Inhalation, Ingestion, and Direct Skin application. Some other methods exist, but these three listed here are the most popularly used methods of application.

The method of application you choose depends basically on the area of action you want the oil to reach and the effect you would need it to produce for you. For some internal problems, you may need to ingest oils to provide you some relive. For a wound, the best method of application should be the skin application. Most of the time, inhalation is the go-to method when you need essential oil to provide emotional relief.

Direct Skin Application

Essential oils are applied directly to the skin from where they can diffuse through the pores and enter

the bloodstream. These oils are known to soothe the skin, the muscular layer, and to open up the pores. Before direct skin application, it is necessary to ascertain the concentration of the essential oil. It might be necessary you dilute them in carrier oils before direct application on the skin. Essential oils fall into three categories,
 which are the neat, the dilute, and the sensitive. Neat simply means that no dilution is necessary. Dilute means that the oils need to be diluted before anyone can use it. Sensitive means that the oil should be diluted before it can be applied on sensitive skin such as an infant's.

Some of these essential oils can be applied to come in direct contact with the skin include massages, bathwater, or facial streams. Just a few drops of your favorite essential oils are enough to produce the desired effect.

Inhalation
Inhalation involves a process of taking the essential oil's smell directly into the nose. This can be done either by releasing drops of the oil on a cloth and sniffing it continuously, mixing with a solvent and spraying around the wall, or by direct inhalation from the bottle. Some of these oils, such as rose otto, are known to produce psychological relaxation when they are inhaled into the lungs. Others provide therapeutic effects that help to balance the emotions of a troubled mind.

After inhalation, some molecules from the oil travel to a major part of the brain known as the limbic brain through the olfactory nerves, where they trigger reactions of relaxation. This limbic part of the brain controls the heart rate, blood pressure, and stress response system.

Ingestion

Ingestion is a rare method of essential oil application and should only be used on prescription. There are a number of essential oils that can be safely ingested, but remember that dosage and quantity of intake also matter. For ingestion, you can add a few drops of the essential oil into an herbal mixture or a drink.

Internal use of Essential Oils

Lots of people interested in essential oils have continued to ask one question: Are these oils safe for use inside of the body? The truth cannot be hidden, which is that some of these oils can produce adverse effects on the body whenever they aren't used properly. There are some factors that can determine your reaction to any oil used on your body, and some of them include your age, any underlying health conditions, and medications. On the side of the oil, it is necessary that you consider some of the following before using them: its chemical concentration, the method, and duration of usage.

If applied internally or externally with the right precautions taken, some essential oils are known to produce rash side effects such as irritation on the skin and burns. The most important point of note when using essential oils internally should be your experience with the oil. Before you are able to use essential oils internally, you must have undergone thorough training with relevant certifications. If you have none of this, then your internal usage of essential oils should depend solely on the advice of someone more experienced, someone like a professional in the field.

Why you will need to take caution with essential oil

The first thing you should know about essential oils is that they are chemicals first before they are oils. Most of them are made of more than ten chemical components that give them powerful qualities and make them perfect for external use only after dilution. Quality essential oils are highly concentrated. They may smell intensely aromatic and very inviting, but they are some of the strongest medicines you can find around.

You might have heard thousands of times before that diluting essential oils in water and taking them in makes them save for ingestion. Well, that is wrong. Remember that these oils, no matter how good they smell, are basically oils, and oil and water do not mix together. Once you take in this mixture of oil and water, the oils are still left as concentrated as ever, floating around in the water. Once they reach your internal system, they begin their attack on the mucus lining your body. This can lead to lots of complications once this process is complete. Some of these include ulceration in the mouth and other severe allergic reactions.

Major Essential oils and associated side effects
It is important that you know some essential oils and the side effects associated with them whenever they are taken internally without any professional advice. Some of these include:

Cinnamon, which is capable of causing irritation on the mucus when it is taken without proper dilution. It can also lead to double vision, nausea, and vomiting.

Lavender oil is feared to negatively affect the sex hormones of males who haven't reached puberty.

Peppermint oil is notorious for causing heartburn when taken internally without proper dilution.

Blending Essential Oils
Essential oils are usually blended before usage for better results. The process of blending oils is quite easy, but there are lots of considerations that you will need to put into place before you start the blending process. The first consideration to make is to ascertain the essential oils that work best when blended. Then you will also want to consider the sequence with which you add each of the oils. The sequencing is capable of affecting the chemical reaction between the oils, and if it turns out to be wrong, the blend won't produce the best results. Some blends are made using just two or three essential oils, while others can be made using up to seven oils. If you can only understand the principle behind the addition of each of the oils, you won't find it hard to create the blends.

Why is it necessary to blend essential oils?
Essential oils are potent on their own, but they perform even better whenever they work in synergy with other oils. All essential oils possess powerful and weak compounds. The powerful compounds are those that work to produce the results we see. The more fragile compounds are those capable of producing adverse effects when used. When

essential oils are blended before usage, one oil is capable of balancing and enhancing the action qualities of the compounds in the other oil, sometimes eliminating any form of adverse reaction.

Understanding Essential Oils Groups
Before you begin to blend essential oils, you have to understand how they are grouped, which are essential oils that share the same traits with each other. These similar traits can be their aromatic qualities, effects they produce when they are used, or any other characteristics you may think will suit you according to your interaction with essential oils.

According to the effects, here are some significant groupings of essential oils.

Calming Effect: Lavender, Geranium, Jasmine, Palmarosa, Sandalwood, Melissa, Bergamot, Mandarin, Ylang Ylang, Neroli.

Detoxifying Effect: Peppermint, Hyssop, Patchouli, Helichrysum, Grapefruit, Lemon, Juniper, Laurel, and thyme.

Anti-Anxiety: Geranium, Lavender. Marjoram, Lemon, Valerian, Chamomile Roman, Sandalwood, Jasmin, Black Pepper, Melissa, and Tangerine.

Energizing Effect: Basil, Grapefruit, Bergamot, Lemongrass, Clary Sage, Eucalyptus, Spearmint, Tea Tree, Ginger, Rosemary.

Creating a blend of essential oils in one group will produce better results. The classification of essential oils, according to their traits, is the most effective method of classification.

Essential Oils Notes

In aromatherapy and the usage of essential oils, one prominent figure is one of the aromatic notes. It is these notes that are used to differentiate one essential oil from the other in terms of how long the aroma will last after usage. The major classifications of notes are the Top, Middle, and Base notes. Most essential oils are characterized mostly by the presence of one-note, but some special ones possess more than one note, which makes them even more appealing.

When essential oils are blended and allowed for a while, you will discover after some time that there will be fluctuation in the strength and aroma of the blend. After a while, the combination stops being as powerful as it used to be. This can easily be attributed to the notes of the various essential oils that make up the blend. Different essential oils have varying levels of volatility, and it is this volatility that affects the rate of evaporation of a particular essential oil. When a blend is created with several essential oils, and one of the oils evaporates, living only the others in the mixture, the blend never remains the same. All of this can only be stopped when the essential oil is stored up in a cool place, to prevent evaporation.

Top Notes: Essential oils characterized by the top notes are those with the smallest molecules. These are most volatile, and it is easier for them to evaporate from an open bottle. Their scents are the first detected in a blend whenever the bottle is opened. Examples include bay, mint, vanilla, rosemary, cypress, yarrow, cardamom, petitgrain, sage, and ravensara essential oils.

Middle Notes: The middle notes can sometimes be referred to as the harmonizers because they serve the purpose of somewhat harmonizing the top notes, and the base notes essential oils. The middle notes can be easily perceived when the top notes fade. They come right after. The middle note essential oils serve to balance the oils and give the blend a form of uniform aroma that makes it smell like one oil. The middle notes essential oils last longer than the top notes and can be perceived about an hour after application. Some examples include rose, black pepper, cinnamon, juniper, myrrh, geranium, cinnamon, myrtle, berry, clove bud, and cedarwood essential oils.

The Base Notes: The base notes have the largest and heaviest molecules making them hardest to evaporate. When applied on a surface, they release their fragrance the slowest, making them last longest in a blend. When used in a blend with essential oils with lower notes, they help to reduce the rate of evaporation and help the aroma of the blend last longer. These kinds of oils are known to provide calming and relaxing sensations. Some examples include frankincense, sandalwood, valerian, copaiba, balsam, patchouli, and vetiver essential oils.

Carrier Oil

Throughout this book, you will come across numerous references to the concept of carrier oils. So the question now is what carrier oils are and how they are necessary for aromatherapy or in the usage of essential oils. Simply put, carrier oils are oils made from plants, and they are used in the production of essential oils blends so that they do not cause damaging reactions.

Most carrier oils used in the production of blends already have their admirable qualities and pleasant aroma before they are added to the blend. Some popular examples of essential oils include vegetable oil, coconut oil, avocado oil e.t.c

How to select a carrier oil for use
When trying to produce a blend of essential oils, you will have to make a selection of carrier oil at some point. It is your selection that determines how good your blend will be and how well the mixture will work. Some of the major criteria in which carrier oils are selected include their aroma, the absorption rate, the skin type of the person who will be using the blend, and the shelf life of the carrier oil.

Why all of these are necessary is because some carrier oils have a strong and distinct aroma that can easily alter the aroma of the other essential oils that may be added to the blend. If that happens, the whole essence of the blend becomes defeated. As for the absorption rate, some carrier oils are known to be easily absorbed into the skin more than others. The better the absorption rate, the better its functionality. Also, considering the skin type of the user is necessary because some sensitive skins can react adversely to some carrier oils. Some carrier oils are known to cause acne, extra oiliness, and skin irritation when they are brought in contact with some skin types. Finally, shelf life. Some essential oils last longer than others without losing their essence, and this, in turn, affects the stability of the blend after a while.

Some Carrier Oils and their Uses

Coconut Oil

The coconut oil is made from the meat of the coconut. The oil has been used as a moisturizer for years and is also known for its antibacterial qualities. The oil has a strong coconut smell and can be applied to the body for its benefits or used carrier oil. Coconut oil is a skin-nourishing oil which makes it very suitable for massage and skincare essential oil blend.

Jojoba Oil

This oil comes from the seeds of the jojoba plant. This oil is more wax than oil, and it is commonly used for massages. Because of its anti-inflammatory qualities, the oil is a go-to option for acne. It is known to closely mimic the activities of the sebum produced on the skin. Jojoba oil easily gets absorbed into the skin pores and is known sometimes to clog them when used in excess quantity. For this quality, it is used in the production of blends used for massages, facial moisturizers, and bath oils.

Apricot Kernel Oil

The apricot kernel oil is produced from apricot seeds, which are also known as kernels. The oil is rich in fatty acids and vitamin E, and it is easily absorbed into the skin. Its aroma is nutty and sweet. The apricot oil is majorly used in the production of essential oil blend used for massaging the skin and in hair care.

Olive Oil

Olive oil is gotten when olives are pressed until the oil oozes out. The oil is major popular for being used by the Jews in the ordination of priests and anointing of new kings as recorded in the Bible. It is also known as a healthy oil used in cooking. Apart from all these, it plays an essential role in aromatherapy, where it is used as a carrier oil

.

Grapeseed Oil
The grapeseed oil is used in the production of blends in aromatherapy. It is referred to it as an all-purpose carrier oil. Its uses vary from massage blends, skincare blends to hair care blends, e.t.c. This oil has a sweet, nutty smell, and it usually leaves a slightly glossy film on the skin.

Diffusers
Simply put, those diffusers are essential hand-in-hand with essential oils. They serve as augmentations to these oils and how they are used. Diffusers can simply be described as devices that break down aromatic compounds and gradually release them into the air until the atmosphere becomes steadily saturated with the sweet-smelling aroma of the used essential oil. Before the arrival of these devices in the aromatherapy market, essential oils were dropped into spray bottles, shaken thoroughly, and sprayed in various corners of the home. Diffusers just make the job easier because they first break down the aromatic compounds before releasing them into the atmosphere, making them last longer in the atmosphere and easier to inhale.

Types of Diffusers
In this book, you are going to come across numerous mentions of the concept of diffusers, so it is wise that you understand the different types of diffusers and how they function. These are the

major ones available to you as a practicing aromatherapist.

Nebulizing Diffusers: These kinds of diffusers are capable of functioning without water or heat. It operates mainly by making use of pressure to diffuse a film of oil into the air.

Ultrasonic or Humidifying Diffusers: These kinds of diffusers break up the essential oils before they are released as a mist into the atmosphere. The essential oil is first mixed with water before it is added into the diffuser. These kinds of diffusers are best for the cold season since they add a moisty and pleasant texture to the dry air. The inner part of these kinds of diffusers is usually lined with plastic, which will require occasional cleaning, so the oily residue doesn't destroy it.

Electric/Heat Diffusers: This diffuser converts electrical energy into heat energy, which helps convert the oil into gas. The only thing with this kind of diffuser is that essential oils tend to lose some of their aromatic qualities when they are heated, so the aroma that is released into the air isn't as concentrated and qualitative as it should be.

Evaporative Diffusers: This one works almost like the electric diffuser, the main difference is that instead of heat, it makes of a fan to turn the oil into gas. Just like in the heat diffuser, the essential oils lose their potency when used in this kind of diffuser.

Benefits of using Diffusers
The question now is, 'Why do you have to use diffusers?' Why not just continue with the old tradition of using spray bottles?

First off, with diffusers, you can use essential oils blends better than you could have done with spray bottles. You can choose a class of oils that perform almost the same function and create a signature blend peculiar to you and your home. With diffusers, everything is automated.

You don't have to keep spraying your home every passing hour. The diffuser does this job for you, slowly releasing the aroma of the essential oil into the air and gradually saturating the atmosphere with it.

Safety Measures with Essential Oils
There are some small procedures that you should take note of if you are going to be using essential oils successfully. First is that if essential oils are to be ingested, make sure that you get recommendations from a professional so that you don't complicate matters for yourself.

When using oils, make sure that they don't come in contact with your eyes.

If you ever ingest any essential oil accidentally, take in any fatty substance or milk to reduce the reaction process in the body.

Make sure to wash your hands after handling essential oils.
Keep the bottle away from the reach of children.

Chapter Three: Basic Essential Oils You Will Need

Essential oils have become something of essential commodities in this modern world, and they serve a variety of purposes, as highlighted in the previous chapter. There are about a hundred essential oils available in the world today, and all of these have special roles they play in different industries such as the perfume production, skincare, and home improvement. But amongst all of these, some essential oils are almost more essential than others, and it is these oils that every practitioner of aromatherapy should have. Most of these have become extremely popular for their relative cheapness, availability, and number of essential qualities they possess. Some of these include:

Lavender Oil
Lavender is so powerful that it is sometimes referred to as the mother of essential oils. It is almost indispensable. Lavender is distilled from the flower spikes of some spices of the lavender plant. Lavender oil is vital in perfume production, in aromatherapy, and skincare.

There are also a variety of other uses for lavender, such as for acne, soothing dry skin, lightening the skin, for dental abscess, and insomnia. Lavender is also vital as an emotional enhancer. It helps to provide calmness and relaxation whenever it is applied to a troubled personality. It was also known for its anti-inflammatory, antifungal, and antiseptic functions.

Rosemary Oil
Rosemary oil is another quite popular essential that you will come across many times in this book. Rosemary receives its name from a Latin term which means 'Dew of the Sea.'

Lots of civilizations in the early world, such as the Egyptians and Greeks, made use of the oil for memory improvement, protection, and wound dressing.
Rosemary oil is essential in aromatherapy to reduce stress and tension levels. It is also known for its respiratory decongestion qualities. When blended with a carrier oil and applied on the hair, rosemary oil is known to improve hair growth and strengthen hair roots. Rosemary oil, when mixed with water, can be made into household fresheners to provide an inviting smell.

Peppermint Oil
Peppermint, as an essential oil, is very much important in dealing with problems of the digestive tract. Peppermint oil has a sharp smell that brings coolness when applied to the body. Its major components are menthol and menthone. In the case of irritable bowel syndrome, nausea, and the common cold, peppermint oil is a go-to solution.

Peppermint oil is also used as a flavoring in foods and drinks. Because of its pleasing scent and its cooling effect on the body, it can be found in some soap and cosmetic products.

Lemon Oil
Lemon oil, as the name implies, is an essential oil that is extracted from the peels of fresh lemon fruits. Lemon oil can be used in different ways, either

applied directly on the skin or inhaled from a cloth or cotton wool.

Lemon oil is known to improve mood and enhance relaxation whenever it is used alongside other cleaning agents. The lemon scent of the oil produces a calm feeling when inhaled.

The pleasant scent is an important commodity in the perfuming industry, where it is blended with other oils to give a distinct smell. Lemon oil can improve the metabolic activities of the body and is also useful in skin routines. This essential oil is important for its antiseptic quality and distinct taste that makes it important as a flavoring agent.

Chamomile Roman Oil
Chamomile oil is produced from different chamomile plants, but the most important and popular amongst this is the chamomile roman oil. The chamomile roman oil is mainly popular for its anti-inflammatory qualities. It also has antibacterial and antiseptic qualities that make it useful in treating burns. Other conditions in which chamomile roman is used include strains, diarrhea, and nausea. The power of chamomile oils has reached the extent where it serves as oil that soothes the body, soul, and spirit. The oil can be used as a calming agent for a troubled mind or a stressed personality.

Thyme Oil
From the name, it is easy to identify the source of this oil, which is the everyday thyme used in cooking. Apart from its importance as a flavoring agent, thyme is also important for its oil. The oil is known for its antifungal, anti-inflammatory, and

antibacterial properties. It is also vital as a preservative in the beauty and food industry.

Research has gone ahead to prove the importance of thyme oil in eliminating bacteria in food and also to improve the health of the heart. When this oil is blended with carrier oils and applied, it is known to be a solution for stubborn acne, respiratory infections, and oral problems.

Tea Tree Oil
Tea tee oil as an essential oil contains the compound terpinene-4-ol, which known for its deadly effect on bacteria, viruses, and fungi. The compound also appears to support the action of white blood cells and helps to boost the immune system. Because of these anti-microbial qualities, it is valued as a treatment for microbial skin infections. Some of the major skin conditions cured by tea tree oil include ringworm, athlete's foot, and candida.

Tea tree oil is also an important ingredient in the production of mouthwashes and bathing lotions. It is also applied in the treatment of insect stings, and its scent is capable of repelling some insects.

Chapter Four: Essential Oils for Health Care

In this chapter, we are going to consider some common essential oils that are used in the health industry. Some significant conditions will be highlighted and explored, and the respective essential oils that can be used to provide relief from them will be given.

Liver Cleanse

Liver cleansing basically involves the detoxification of the organ. Some of the most common essential oils that can be used for liver cleansing include rosemary oil, peppermint oil, and lemon essential oil. All of these work together to reduce the toxic materials lodged in the liver. The peppermint oil works to facilitate lymph drainage.

To prepare the therapy, add few drops of peppermint, rosemary, and lemon essential oil into one spoon of lemon juice. Pour the mixture into a glass of water. Gulp down the whole mixture in one sip. You can do this once every day of the week.

In the case of a severe hangover, liver cleansing may help to relieve the feeling of dizziness and nausea. The essential oils that can be used for this are the ginger essential oil and the lemon essential oil. You can prepare the mixture with a spoonful of fresh lemon juice squeeze, some drops of ginger essential oil and lemon essential oil. All of this while be diluted in a glass of water and taken down in one whole gulp. You can use this procedure whenever you find yourself struggling with hangovers.

Stomach Ache
There are essential oils that are known to help alleviate the pains of stomach aches. The recipes and mixture can be used on anyone, both kids and adults. The essential oil mostly used for the relief of stomach pain is lavender. It is usually described as an analgesic oil which helps to relieve pains. Another such is the geranium essential oils, which create balance in the body and possess anti-inflammatory qualities. Peppermint essential oil acts as an antispasmodic agent and a stimulant. The last ingredient on the list is the rosemary oil, which is an anti-septic agent.

To produce the mixture, add three drops of lavender, geranium, peppermint, and rosemary to two spoonful of vegetable oils. Mix with a spoon and use the combination to massage the abdomen in a clockwise direction.

In the case of severe indigestion that is causing pain, you can use peppermint oil as a remedy. The menthol contained in the mixture is known to halt nausea and improve the action of the circulatory system. Get a clean cloth or a ball of cotton wool. Pour three drops of the essential peppermint oil on the cloth. Keep it placed under the nose, but prevent contact with your skin. Take in the aroma slowly for about 3 minutes.

Muscle Pain
There are a number of essential oil that are useful in fighting muscle pain. Some of these include peppermint, helichrysum oil, and marjoram oil. The menthol in peppermint is important because it creates a cooling effect on sores and painful muscles. It is necessary for its analgesic effect.

Helichrysum helps to produce relief for muscle spasms and inflammations. Marjoram oil relieves muscle tension and spasm. Each of these oils can be used separated or can be combined as a mixture.

These oils for relieving muscle tension can sometimes irritate the skin, so you should mix them with carrier oils to dilute before usage.

To create a mixture, add about ten drops of your selected essential oil. Add in the carrier oil and mix vigorously. Roll the bottle on your palm so the mixture can achieve an even consistency.

Use the mixture to massage the muscle group where you feel pains. Do well to press your hands in a kneading motion so that the oils can penetrate the skin and produce a release of tension. Only ensure that the oils are well diluted to prevent skin irritation. Essential oils for muscle massage are best applied using roll-on bottles.

Essential oils can also be added to bathwater to loosen stiff muscles. After mixing your select oils with the carrier oil, add some drops of the mixture to a bucket filled with water. Stir with your hands until the oil spreads evenly. Use this to bath slowly or immerse your body in the mixture for about 10 minutes.

In the case of muscle overuse, which can lead to stiffness and an abundance of lactic acid, a mixture of drops of lavender oil, scots pine, and eucalyptus essential oil should provide you with relief. Blend all of these with a carrier oil using the same direction outlined above. Gently massage the affected area with the mixture.

Cuts, Burns and Bruises
If you end up with a cut or a burn, your number one priority should be protecting the wound to prevent infection. One way to do about this, apart from the conventional medical procedures, is the topical application of essential oils on the affected areas.

Some essentials oils are known to provide protection and healing qualities to burns and cuts. Some of the most notable ones that are used for this purpose include eucalyptus, lavender, oregano, sage, and peppermint. Some of these can be included in your first aid kit for easy accessibility.

Before applying these essential oils, it is necessary to ensure that the wounds aren't too severe. Essential oils are only necessary for minor cuts and bruises that may not require serious medical help. In the case that medical care isn't needed, then you can go ahead with this procedure.

The first thing to do is to clean up the cut or bruise with clean water. Applying essential oil on a dirty wound might end up
complicating the issue.
Hydrogen peroxide, when applied, can help you better in getting rid of the dirt or possible infestation.

With the wound clean, add drops of your select essential oil on it. Making use of cotton wool, spread the oil evenly on the top of the wound. Wrap it around with a bandage and ensure to repeat the procedure at least twice per day and change the bandage.

Another way to go about applying your select oil on the wound is to make a mixture with water by adding some drops into a bowl. Stir and mix with a spoon. Soak a clean cloth in the mixture and squeeze over the wound until drops land on the cut. Repeat this until all the water I have gone.

Helichrysum and marigold essential oils are perfect for bruises because of their anti-inflammatory qualities. Blend drops of these oils with a carrier oil of your choice and apply on the bruise twice per day.

Common Cold and Flu
Just like with the treatment of wounds and bruises, you must understand the severity of your cold before you decide to make use of essential oils to start treatment. Essential oils can be used to provide temporary relief before professional medical help can be gotten. Some of the oils that can be used for this purpose include eucalyptus, thyme, douglas fir, rosemary, and lemon.

The first method is to add drops of your chosen essential oils into a pail of hot, steaming water. Bend over and cover up your head with a thick cloth so that all the stream goes directly into your nose. Maintain the position for more than three minutes. You can make use of a mixture of eucalyptus, which is known to ease nasal congestion, chest coughs and stuffy nose, and thyme, which is known for its antispasmodic properties.

The oils can also be sniffed directly from the bottle or dropped on balls of cotton wool or handkerchiefs to be sniffed continuously. Ensure not to inhale large amounts of oil, because this is known sometimes to cause headaches, nausea, or dizziness.

In the case of a sore throat caused by the common cold or flu, use echinacea essential oil in warm water to help provide relief. The mixture is produced simply by adding five drops of the essential oil into a glass of warm water. After stirring the mixture and spreading the oil evenly throughout the glass, take in a large amount into your mouth and gargle with it. Do this twice every day until you notice total relief.

Oral Health
Essential oils are one quick way to improve oral health and prevent consistent visits to the dentist. The best among these are oils, which are known to have antibacterial qualities. Essential oils used to maintain oral health can kill bacteria, eliminate bad breath, and strengthen the dental cavities.

Two essential oils that can serve this purpose include seabuckthorn oil and rose oil. Rose oil is quite expensive, so you may want to go for the seabuckthorn oil. Other oils you can add to the mixture include peppermint, oregano, thyme, tea tree, and clove essential oils.

The blend can be produced by adding three drops of all of these oils into a carrier oil to dilute them. Make the mixture in a dark-colored bottle because the blend will be used more than once, so you will need to preserve it.

Add drops of the blend to your toothbrush alongside your regular paste before brushing. You can also take a swipe of it at the tip of your finger and use it in massaging your gums.

In the event of a dental abscess, pour drops of chamomile roman oil on cotton wool and drag it gently over the abscess. Also, mix the oil with a carrier and rub directly on the abscess at least once per week, apart from the normal cotton wool procedure.

Headaches
In the case of a mild headache, there a variety of essential oils you can use to provide some relief for yourself. One precaution that should be taking with the usage of essential oils for headaches is to note that the oils don't have the same effect for everyone. For some people, the odor of these oils may turn out to be too powerful and cause even more headaches. However, for more people, essential oils produce great relief from headaches or migraines. Remember to ensure that your headache isn't too severe or the type that may require professional medical attention.

Your choice of essential oil will depend on the kind of headache you are experiencing. These are some of the most common ones that are used for different severity levels of headaches.

Peppermint essential oil is best used in the case of a tension headache when it feels like there is a tightening sensation around the head. Peppermint oil is known to reduce tension when applied anywhere on the body. You can create your blend by adding a few drops of the oil to your chosen carrier oil. Mix the blend well and use it to massage your forehead, your neck, and shoulders.

In the case of headaches caused mostly by stress, the essential oils mostly used are lavender, frankincense, and Citrus. All of these oils are known to reduce the stress level of the body by stabilizing the blood pressure. Your choice of essential oil depends entirely on your favorite. Take a bottle of your selected essential oil and inhale deep breaths until you feel the odor cursing through your body. You can release drops of the oil on a tissue paper or handkerchief to be inhaled continuously for a more extended period.

In the case of a mild migraine, the essential oil you can use is lavender. At this point, you will notice that lavender serves a lot of purposes. That is the beauty of this oil. You can sniff straight from the bottle, or you can a few drops to your body lotion and apply at strategic parts of your head such as the jaws, the temples, and the back of your neck.

Heartburn
Whenever you experience that burning sensation in your chest after eating a meal, don't worry about finding medications. You can use some essential oils to provide relief for yourself before you can get professional help. Some of the major oils you can use in the case of heartburn include:

Lemon oil has properties capable of neutralizing the heartburn-causing acid in the stomach. The oil is an alkaline one with antibacterial qualities capable of wiping off bacteria existing in the digestive system. Since heartburn is known to start up after some meals, you can add drops of your lemon essential oil into a glass of warm water and gulp it down some minutes before you start eating. This should prepare your body and digestive system for what is to come.

The ginger essential oil can also be used because of its anti-inflammatory and antibacterial qualities. The oil helps to reduce the production of acids in the stomach, thereby reducing the probability of heartburns occurring.

To use ginger oil, add a few drops of it to your herbal tea and sip in the morning or before any heartburn-causing meal. In the event that you also notice some bloating in your stomach, dilute drops of the oil in a carrier oil and use it to massage your chest and abdominal areas.

Finally, you can also make use of orange essential oil, which contains properties that help to reduce acid reflux by preventing muscle spasms. You can add drops of this essential oil into a warm glass of water or herbal tea and gulp it down before meals.

Palpitations
Research has shown that essential oils play an essential role in the control and reduction of blood pressure. But they should be used in the event of mild blood pressure. Sometimes your blood pressure can get so high that you may need to seek out professional help for the right advice. Essential oils can be used to produce temporary relief before you can see your doctor and lay a complaint.

There are several essential oils that can be used for heart palpitations. Some of these include citronella, bergamot, jasmine, helichrysum, lime, sweet marjoram, yarrow, clary sage, and frankincense. Each of these essential oils can be used alone, or they can be mixed to form blends before being applied. One way this blend can be created is by adding drops of lavender, frankincense, and clary sage into a carrier oil such as jojoba oil. Mix all of these by stirring. You can inhale the mixture occasionally and make use of it to massage your thoracic region.

Whitlows
Whitlow is a lesion that develops around the fingernails, causing swelling and pains. It is majorly caused by contact with a person infected with the herpes simplex one virus. Some standard drugs can be prescribed whenever a person develops whitlow. But essential oils serve an easily accessible home-made remedy.

Garlic oil is known to have antimicrobial properties that make it very useful in battling whitlow because of its antimicrobial properties. There is also a high quantity of allicin and ajoene in garlic essential oil. Both of these contain antiviral qualities that help to fight the herpes virus that causes whitlow.

To treat, soak cotton wool in essential garlic oil and leave for some time. Squeeze the cotton wool and allow drops of the oil to fall on the whitlow, then dab gently on the surface. This procedure can also be produced with peppermint oil, which produces a cooling effect and helps to reduce the burning sensation felt on the finger. Apply these oils about thrice each day until the growth begins to dry up.

Anal Fissures
Anal fissure in adults is caused whenever there is a tear in the anal canal of a person. This tear can lead to lots of pain and infection if proper precaution isn't taken. Feces sometimes get stuck in the fresh wound and lead to constant itching and irritation. This anal fissure has to be treated quite carefully, or

the wounds will only widen and cause more irritation and pain. Sometimes it is best to consult with your doctor or a professional before you begin to use essential oils on your anal fissures. If you are cleared to use essential oils, then these should help out.

For this purpose, the two most used essential oils include yarrow and witch hazel oil. These two have astringent agents that help to constrict the flow of blood and reduce bleeding from anal fissures. Calendula and chamomile essential oils are used for their anti-inflammatory quality. They are used to keep the wound clean while the anal canal heals.

To produce the perfect blend for this, add drops of calendula, chamomile, yarrow, and witch hazel essential oils into a bowl of warm water. Select a bowl you can easily sit in without feeling uncomfortable. Stir the mixture and sit in it for about ten minutes. Once you step out, use a clean cloth to dab the fissures and keep it dry for about an hour.

Other essential oils that are used for anal fissures include lavender and lemon, which can be dropped on cotton wool and applied on the open fissure after dilution with a carrier oil. Other essential oils that can be used for this purpose include frankincense, cinnamon bark, clove, peppermint, and tea tree essential oils.

Black eyes
Black eyes are characterized by dark circles underneath the eyes that are caused as a result of sleep, aging, and extreme stress. These dark circular lines appearing under the eyes can lead to disfiguration of the face making an individual look

unattractive. These circles can be gotten rid of using essential oils that are blended with carrier oils.

Essential oils used in treating black eyes are mostly those oils known to be very healthy for the skins with anti-inflammatory properties, which can reduce unnecessary growths on the skin. Some of these oils include chamomile, rose geranium, lavender, and cypress oils.

Cypress oil is always a wonder worker in the elimination of dark circles underneath the eyes. It works by dealing with excess body fluids flooding the area and causing puffiness. Cypress essential oil is mixed with shea butter before usage and applied under the eyes overnight for concentrated attention.

Lavender is mixed with a carrier oil to create a blend which is used to massage underneath the eyeballs. Lavender oil, when applied under the eyes, is known to induce sleep and work as an anti-oxidant agent on the skin in that area.

Rose geranium oil is another very important essential oil for treating black eyes. The oil works to reduce puffiness of skin when applied on any part of the skin, and this makes it perfect for treating black eyes. It also has some anti-aging qualities that help to mildly replenish old skin and create a feeling of elasticity. A blend is produced by adding three drops of rose geranium to a teaspoon of aloe vera. This mixture is used to massage underneath the eyes every day before sleep.

Bleeding
Essential oils can also be used to treat wounds and reduce bleeding. They are very useful in enhancing

the healings of these wounds. In the case of a really deep wound, it is necessary that you visit your doctor for proper treatment. These oils are mostly used whenever there is a small and minor wound.

Before essential oils are used on wounds, it is necessary that the wound be cleaned with warm water and a saline solution using a clean cloth or cotton wool. After the wound has been cleaned thoroughly, then you can begin the application of any of these oils.
Frankincense is important for the replenishing and rejuvenation of damaged skins. Add three drops of the oil to another carrier oil to create a blend. Rub the blend over a clean wound and allow it rest for about ten minutes. The process will help in the development of cells responsible for the reduction of bleeding.

Rosemary oil is known to protect the wound and prevent the invasion of infections. Add three drops of the oil to a carrier oil and rub the blend over the wound with a clean cloth or a ball of cotton wool.

Finally, a blend of lavender, tea tree and chamomile german oil mixed with a carrier oil. This blend can be applied to the wound.

Boils
Some essential oils can be used in skincare and eliminating blemishes from the skin. This makes them good for taking care of boils, rashes, and acne. Boils can be treated by directly spreading the undiluted oils on the top of the boils or by diluting and applying the blend over the boil continuously over some time. The application of essential oils does not only help to dissolve the boils, but also

prevents its spread to other parts of the body. Two major examples of essential oils that can be used for this purpose include roman chamomile and tea tree.

To begin treatment, release two drops of roman chamomile and tea tree oils on the boil. Dip a clean towel in hot water and squeeze. Check that the towel isn't too hot before placing it on the boil. Allow it to rest on the top of the boil until the towel returns to room temperature. Repeat this procedure about 2 to 3 times daily until the boil disappears.

In the cases of a mild boil, you can add two drops of lavender and thyme oil in a warm water and use a clean cloth to dab the top of the boil.

Blisters
There are several ways in which blisters can be treated to reduce the pain they cause on the skin. But when essential oils are applied to them, they become less painful and heal quite faster. Also, essential oils protect the top of the blister and prevent infection. There are several essential oils that are used in treating blisters some of which include peppermint, lavender and tea tree oils.

All of these are in popular use because of their antimicrobial, antifungal and anti-inflammatory qualities. Tea tree oil is specifically used for its antimicrobial quality. It is applied as a disinfectant to the skin. Peppermint oil on the hand is very good for treating cold sores that appear on the skin.

To treat, apply drops of peppermint and tea tree oil on the blister and spread gently over the surface so that you don't break the surface of the blister. Other essential oils that can be to treat blisters include lemon oil, frankincense and aloe vera essential oils.

Catarrh
Catarrh is basically characterized by the congestion of the nasal cavity. Essential oils known for their decongesting capabilities are usually applied to provide relief to the nasal cavity. Some of the oils include cedarwood, eucalyptus and ginger oils. They can be added to steam inhalers or used in baths to provide some form of relief.

Add streaming hot water into a bowl and add drops of your selected essential oils to create a mixture. Bow your head and place a thick blanket from your head down to the bowl so that the stream rises directly into your nostrils. Also, you can make a blend of tea tree oil, rosemary and thyme with a carrier and rub it over your chest.
Some other essential oils that can be used in treating catarrh include lavender oil, cajuput and niaouli.

Chapter Five: Essential Oils for Children

As has already been established in this book, essential oils are valuable in various aspects of life, and this extends into childcare. Some essential oils can be applied to children in various growing stages of their lives to help them have a successful transition into the next phase. Note that when using essential oils on children, the dosage should never be overlooked. Also, understand the essential oils needed for any child at a particular age. These oils are required in order to help them cope with the stress of school, to promote sleeping habits, and protect them from microbial infection.

In this chapter, we are going to consider the various growing stages in children and the most common essential oils needed for each stage, how to use them, and the reason they are needed during that growing phase.

Essential Oils for Baby/Toddler Phase

In the baby phase, the use of essential oil is necessary to produce a feeling of relaxation and calmness in a child. One major precaution you should take before making use of essential oil on a baby is to ensure that it is well diluted with a carrier oil before application. If a mistake is made, the damage might be permanent, since the baby's skin isn't developed enough to protect itself. Also, never use essential oils internally on babies. You can allow them to inhale or use on the skin once in a while but never use it orally. Babies younger than four months old should never be exposed to them, except when sprinkled for its aromatic effect.

Another consideration to be made is to ensure that you don't get to overuse essential oils on your baby. This can lead to a phenomenon known as systematic sensitization, which will generally result in the inability to use essential oils on the baby.

Essential oils are powerful and very effective when used on babies. Still, one question you should ask yourself before using essential oils on your baby is, "What other option do I have if I decide not to use essential oils?" You will be shocked by the number of other alternatives you have at your disposal.

Safety precautions for using essential oils on babies
Before you begin to use any essential oil on your baby, here are some safety measures that you can put in place to make the process a smooth one.

Introduce your baby to one oil per time so that they don't become overwhelmed by the different aromas, which can cause a sickening effect.

The first and most important is to consult a health professional before you start using these oils, especially if the baby is sick or has some underlying health challenge that may cause a reaction and lead to complications.

Essential oils are highly concentrated and should never be inhaled by babies under four months old for no reason.

Make use of a diffuser in or around the crib to infuse the desired scent around the air in the nursery. Don't add in too much oil so that the air doesn't become too dense with the aroma.

When essential oils are added to baths, take care to ensure that your baby does not splash. When they do this, they are prone to have some of the oil go into their mouth or splash into their eyes.

Introduce your baby to the oil as gradually as possible. Start by applying the oil on your body before coming in contact with them so that they get used to it before you start to use it on them.

Ensure that the oil is well diluted before you start to use it entirely on the baby. A small test you can perform is a spot test where you expose a part of the baby's body to the diluted oil to check for reactions. If there is no reaction after some minutes, then it means that the oil is now safe for usage on the baby's skin.

Essential oils for babies between the ages of 4 months to 1-year-old
One must take caution while making use of essential oils for babies that fall within this age range. Most times, it is hard to tell what is making your baby cry, and you may find yourself jumping into conclusion and making deductions. Sometimes these deductions may be wrong, and other times you may find out that they are right. So the first step here is to find whatever it is that is making your baby uncomfortable. Once that is settled, you can then find which oil will be perfect for solving the problem. That being said, here are some of how essential oils can be used to help your baby.

Baby Skin Massage
The benefits of baby massage are enormous for your baby, both on the physical and the emotional level. First off, massages are a way of

communicating love to your baby since you can't necessarily talk to them. The strokes and skin to skin contact that come with baby massages are important for awakening the emotional part of that child. At this point in its life, touch and food are the only languages that the baby understands. Touch is known to facilitate the production of oxytocin, which is generally referred to as the 'Love Hormone.'

Before you begin to consider a massage session for your baby, be sure that the baby is feeling well, without any symptoms of stress or fever. The best place to place your baby during massage is on a large bed or on the floor, to prevent any likeliness of a fall. Take off any pieces of jewelry on your fingers and cut off extra-long fingernails that cut the baby's skin. Finally, your hands should be clean before you start the process to prevent any infections.

So which oil is the safest oil to use while massaging your baby? There are several essential oils that can be used in baby massage. The one you select depends solely on the purpose of the massage or if your baby is battle with any health challenge. Some of these essential oils include:

Lavender Oil: Lavender is known to help users handle pain better, and this also extends to usage in babies. Studies have shown that lavender oil can be used to treat pain in babies when the right points are massaged. Studies from NCBI have discovered that babies who inhale lavender oil are more prone to cope with pain than when they are left without it.

Chamomile Oil: When a few drops of this are added to baby bathwater, it is believed to relieve restlessness and sleep.

Sunflower Oil: Sunflower is mostly used as a carrier oil to dilute more concentrated oils before they are used on the baby's body. The oil contains a high quantity of linoleic acid, which makes it perfect for use on the baby's body.

In creating the blend to be used on the babies, one thing you should pay close attention to is dosage. The quantity of essential oil used on the baby should be about one-tenth of that used on an adult. A well-mixed essential oil blend, when used on a baby's skin, is capable of reducing the symptoms of skin inflammation, rashes, eczema, and cradle cap. There is also an overall calming effect on the nerves.

To produce a blend, add one drop of lavender and chamomile oil to three teaspoons of the carrier oil. The quantity to be used for the massage session depends solely on the size of the baby.

Diaper Rash
A diaper rash can be an unbearable torment for your baby. This is why you will need to act to get rid of it before it develops into something worse. There are other ways in which diaper can be cured, such as the use of powder, lotions, and creams, but some of these might only expose the baby to more skin irritation. This is one reason why essential oils come in handy for this purpose. Some of the commonly used essential oils include lavender, known for its disinfectant qualities and its ability to hasten the healing process. Lemon essential oil is another good option with antiseptic qualities that can help halt growing symptoms of diaper rash.

To deal with diaper rash, add drops of chamomile and lavender essential oils to a small bowl of warm water. Mix them thoroughly and allow it to rest for a while. Pour the mixture through a filter paper so that the oil droplets can be sieved out before usage. At this point, you have a clear combination, free from droplets of essential oils. Dip a ball of cotton wool and use it to wipe the rashes gently.

You can also create a blend of jojoba oil, aloe vera gel, and tamanu oil. After mixing thoroughly, take a little of the blend and rub it thoroughly between your palms and rub your palms over the sore areas of your baby's buttocks.

Coconut oil can also be applied to affected areas to soothe the pain. Coconut oil should not be used in large quantities, and usage should be stopped if the baby shows any signs of sensitivity to it. Proper monitoring should be employed to check for irritations and reactions.

Baby Coughs and Cold
It is terrible to watch a baby suffer from colds and coughs and not have anything to do to bring it relief. This is a point where essential oils like cajuput, cypress, ravensara, and fragonia essential come to play. Some of these essential oils can be applied to provide relief for your baby until you get professional help if the symptoms don't stop. You can make use of the ravensara oil, by adding two drops of it into steaming hot water and placing the bowl close to your baby's crib. There should be maximum observation so that your baby doesn't move towards the water and get burnt. The steam rising from the water will fill the air around the crib and find its way into your baby's nostrils to help clear the airways.

Another wonderful option you can explore is to add drops of ravensara, lavender, thyme, peppermint, fragonia into a carrier oil and mix to form a blend. Pour a drop of this blend on a ball of cotton wool and place it away from the baby's head where the smell can reach him. Be alert so that the baby doesn't wake up and take the wool into its mouth. If possible, find something small you can enclose the cotton wool in so that the baby's hands won't be able to reach it. The blend can be placed in a diffuser and left overnight in the baby's room.

Early Teething
The teething stage in a baby usually starts between the ages of 4 to 7 months. Two oils are used during this stage to help the baby. They include Chamomile and Lavender.

Chamomile is the more popular oil used for this purpose because of its sedative effect. Its nontoxicity is also another reason why it is a go-to option. To make use of this oil, add two drops of it into a vaporizer containing water. Place the vaporizer in the room overnight so that the baby inhales the smell. Alternatively, you can create a blend containing two drops of chamomile oil and one tablespoon of carrier oil. This blend can be used to massage the jawline of the baby.

Lavender, just like chamomile, is nontoxic for babies, with natural antiseptic qualities. It also possesses sedative qualities that help to relieve pain. To use, make a blend of two drops with a carrier oil and use to massage the baby's jawline.

To Prevent Restlessness and Enhance Sleep

Restlessness and lack of sleep in babies can be caused by several reasons. It could be that the baby is sick, uncomfortable in a sleeping position, or just can't sleep.

For the latter, essential oils can do the trick of providing sleep. One easy solution is to add drops of chamomile and lavender to warm water and place the bowl somewhere in the room. You can also place in a vaporizer so the baby can inhale.

Essential oils for Children

For Insomnia

Insomnia can develop in a child for a variety of reasons, most of which include pure restlessness, stress, and anxiety from schoolwork or relationships with peers. Of course, there are a variety of ways in which you can handle insomnia in your children, depending on the age, but some of these will require that you get professional help and do away with some money. On the other hand, essential oils provide one easy and free way to cure this plague.

When trying to help a child overcome sleeplessness, one major thing that you should try to introduce in the child is relaxation and relief. These can be achieved by bathing them at night, giving a warm cup of tea before bed, or a short story time to allow the mind to wander away until it finds rest. Essential oils can serve as worthy augmentations to all of these. Some major essential oils you can use to help you cure insomnia in your children include chamomile roman, mandarin, and lavender.

Add drops of any of the above listed essential oils to a carrier oil and create a dilute blend. Add one to five drops of the blend to bathwater, depending on the age.

For children older than ten years old, you can use any of the following essential oils to create a blend: Frankincense, Mandarin, Geranium, or Clary sage. Add drops of any of these essential oils with a carrier oil and make a blend that can either be added to bathwater or used for a massage session before bed.

For Body Aches and Pain
Pain or aches in children are mostly caused due to overuse or overworked muscles. The three essential oils used for this are lavender, rosemary, and cypress.

Produce a blend by adding three drops of all these oils to three teaspoons of carrier oil and mix with your finger. Allow the child to take a bath and massage the point where the pain seems to be emanating from.

For Constipation
Essential oils you can use are Rosemary, Mandarin, Lemon, and Geranium oils. Produce a blend by adding two drops of all these oils to a carrier oil and mix. Rub the blend on your palm and massage the abdominal section thoroughly the last thing before bed.

For Measles
The essential oils used in this case include cypress, ravensara, lavender, geranium, chamomile german, and palmarosa oils. Make a blend with three drops

of any of the oils with a carrier oil. Add drops of the blend to a bowl of water. Dip a sponge into the mixture and use the dab around the skin of the child.

You can also add chamomile or lavender to a bottle of calamine lotion. Add 3 drops of the essential oil and allow it to vaporize continuously in the room where your child stays.

Whooping Cough

In the case of whooping cough in children, you can make use of the following essential oils: Eucalyptus, cinnamon, cypress, thyme, geranium, peppermint, and lavender.

Eucalyptus oil is used because of its close association with afflictions of the respiratory tracts like sinusitis and bronchitis. A lot of medications prescribed for coughs have the oil in them because of its renowned quality of dealing with congestion in the nasal cavity. Add ten drops of eucalyptus oil to a bowl of hot water and allow your child to inhale the mixture three times every day until you begin to notice relief.

Cinnamon oil, on the other hand, acts as an antibacterial agent that inhibits the action of pathogens that find their way into the respiratory. It reduces their reproduction and prevents them from spreading further into the respiratory system. Add five drops of cinnamon oil to a bowl of hot water and have your child inhale the steam into the nostrils.

Cypress oil contains camphene, a molecule known to help reduce respiratory congestion when inhaled. Thyme oil is known for its antimicrobial quality in dealing with respiratory conditions. Peppermint oil contains menthol, which, when inhaled, provides relief for the respiratory tract.

Essential oils for cough can be used with on the skin for constant inhalation, added to hot water and inhaled, used in a diffuser, and released into the air or added into bath water to provide relief. Drops of the essential oils can be added to a ball of cotton wool to be sniffed at intervals, or this can also be done straight from the bottle.

To produce a blend for whooping cough, add 5 drops each of cypress, peppermint, cinnamon, and eucalyptus oil to a carrier oil to dilute the oils. Add drops of the blend to a bowl of hot water and place the bowl close to the child's bed. The blend can be rubbed on the palms and used to massage the thoracic cavity of the child. This should be repeated at least twice every day.

For Ringworm
The most commonly used essential oils for treating ringworm in children include tea tree, lavender, manuka, frankincense, palmarosa, and oregano. All of these are wonderful choices because of their antimicrobial qualities that inhibit fungal activities on the skin.

To treat, add undiluted drops of any of the essential oils listed above and spread it over the surface of the ringworm formation. Do this twice every day until you begin to notice the ringworm drying on the skin. Blend three drops of oregano, tea tree, thyme, and mauka oils with a carrier oil. Rub the blend over the cleared surface to prevent the fungi from redeveloping on the surface.

For Athlete's Foot
The most commonly used essential used for treating athlete's foot are peppermint, eucalyptus, lavender, tea tree, and lemon oil. Create a blend by adding one drop of tea tree oil, one drop of lavender, two drops of lemon, two of peppermint and two of eucalyptus oil to a carrier oil like jojoba oil. Wash the infected area thoroughly and apply the blend twice per day. Keep the area open and dry while the oil acts.

Chapter Six: Essential oils for Skin Care

Essential oils provide lots of benefits when they are used on the skin. For one thing, their antiseptic and anti-bacterial qualities are two properties that make them valuable in the inhibition of microbial activities and the enhancement of skin beauty and care. Essential oils also have a way of making the skin tighter and giving new life to the pores underneath the topmost skin layer so that they stay open and allow for the release of sweat in sufficient quantity.

Most first-time users of essential oils for skincare often ask why the option should be chosen over the traditional everyday skincare process using cosmetics products. First, essential oils are more natural than these manufactured products, and this makes them safer for use on the body. Most of the cosmetic products that are used for skincare are loaded with preservatives capable of negatively affecting sensitive skin. All of these go to prove that using essential oils for your skincare routine is your best option. Plus, the results are always marvelous and unbelievable. Truly, essential oils are a gift from nature, and you should maximize them.

Essential oils for Face Masks

Face masks are used every day in the beauty routine, and they work lots of magic. The secret that most people don't know is that you can improve your face masks by adding essential oils to them. The process of making them is both fun and easy to do, and they produce better results than the normal clay face masks. Here are some mixtures you can try on your skin.

The exfoliating face mask
The exfoliating face mask is used to get rid of dead skin cells lying on the face and help the face achieve a smooth feel and texture. Two essential oils used in producing this face mask are chamomile and lemon oil. Chamomile oil makes it easier to scrub off dead skin cells, and lemon oil allows the mixture to circulate freely over the skin surface. Other ingredients need for this include fresh yogurt, vinegar, and salt.

To produce the mixture, add one tablespoon of yogurt, a drop of chamomile and lemon oil, half teaspoon of vinegar, and a pinch of salt. Mix thoroughly with your fingers. Apply the mixture over your face and allow the mixture to rest for about 30 minutes. Rinse off with warm water.

The Oil Control Mask
The oil control mask is used to control the quantity of sebum secreted by the oil glands under the skin. Ingredients to be used in producing this face mask include rhaussol clay, geranium oil, aloe vera, and water. To produce the mixture, add two tablespoons of clay, one tablespoon of aloe vera, three drops of water, and a drop of geranium oil. Mix the ingredients thoroughly with your fingers and apply all over the face. Allow it to rest on the face until it dries. You can then rinse off with warm water.

Another face mask you will enjoy using to remove excess oil from your face is the bergamot face mask. The blend is created by adding 4 drops of lavender, 2 drops of bergamot, 2 drops of clary sage and 2 tablespoons of cornmeal to a quarter glass of water.

Mix the blend with your finger until a consistent paste form in the bowl. Apply the mixture to your face in gentle circular motions until it is all over your face. Allow the mixture to remain on your face until it dries, then rinse off with warm water. Use a clean towel to wipe your face.

Moisturizing Face Mask

This face mask is best used on a dry face to add some of the moisture to it. The two essential oils used for this are orange essential oil and lemon essential oil. These two oils are known for their hydrating quality and the amount of vitamin C they contain, which is responsible for healthy skin.

One other ingredient needed to produce the blend is mashed avocado. After it has been mashed, you can add 3 drops of the two essential oils and mix thoroughly. Apply the mixture on the face and allow it to rest for about 30 minutes, after which you wash off with warm water.

Facial steaming using essential oils

Facial steaming involves exposing the surface of the face to steam from hot water. This steam goes to melt dirt in various forms that lie on the surface of the facial skin, thereby opening the pores of the skin and providing a healthy skin surface. The steam method of facial cleansing is quite easy to carry out. It has been discussed several times in this book. It involves placing the face over rising steam so that there is direct, undisturbed contact. For better results, essential oils are added to the water before the process begins.

Facial steaming cleaning should not be used by people with sensitive skin or people with acne. There might be complications along the way.

If you have none of these conditions, another thing to consider should be the right essential oil to use for the procedure. Some oils are more suited for some skin types than others, especially for this procedure.

For the normal skin that isn't too oily or too dry, the most recommended essential oils include lemon, cedarwood, lavender, fennel, jasmine, and rosemary. All of these oils are known to work in normal skin conditions and produce the desired results of freshness and cleanness without doing anything extra.

The most recommended essential oils to use on dry skin include chamomile german, chamomile roman, cypress, bergamot, frankincense, grapefruit, and palmarosa. These oils are known to open up the skin pores and improve the production of sebum by the sebaceous gland under the skin. When used consistently, they help the skin achieved an oilier texture while eliminating dryness.

For oily skin, the best oils to use include eucalyptus, immortelle, lemongrass, and juniper berry. When used in the right quantity, these oils are known to reduce the production of sebum and its oiliness from spreading over the surface of the skin.

Add 2 to 3 drops of your select essential oil to a bowl of steaming water. Place your head over the bowl so that the steam comes directly towards your face. Use a thick cloth to prevent the steam from spreading out and not reaching your face. Stay that way for about 10 minutes. Use a clean cloth to wipe your face.

Facial Toner with Essential oils
If you notice that your face is usually aging, and a kind of tiredness and dullness is gathering over its surface, then you will benefit immensely from the use of facial toner. Adding essential oils will provide you with better results. There are lots of improvements to texture, color tone, and smoothness that can be achieved on the face when a facial toner is used.

One of such toners you can create is the aloe vera facial toner whose principal ingredient is aloe vera with lime essential oil as the only oil added to the blend. Aloe vera in the mixture provides hydration, while lime is needed for its exfoliating quality. The blend is made by mixing aloe vera and lime oil and applying all over the face, as explained in other processes.

Another powerful toner is the one made with rosemary oil, lemon oil, cornmeal, and almond meal. This blend also works wonders on dry skin with dark patches. It stimulates the production of sebum and tightens the skins, thereby removing dark patches and lines underneath the eyes. The blend is produced by adding one tablespoon of cornmeal, one tablespoon of almond meal, three drops of lemon and rosemary essential oils. Apply the mixture on the face and allow it to dry, then clean up with warm water.

The last toner is produced using the yarrow essential oil. This toner is perfect for oily skin, to regulate the secretion of sebum on the face. The blend is produced by adding three tablespoons of witch hazel with a drop of a weak acid such as boric acid. Add water and the essential oils and keep in a bottle to be stored in a cool place. Use a ball of cotton wool to apply on the skin occasionally.

Essential oils for wrinkling and aging skin

It is no secret that all of us, as humans are going to lose the youthful beauty and attractiveness we once possessed and cherished. But even with this knowledge, lots of people are willing to go to any length to ensure that they keep themselves young, even going as far as spending thousands of dollars on getting work done on their bodies. Sometimes these procedures work and produce brilliant results that make their peers burn with envy, but the truth is that everything unnatural comes with a price to pay. A lot of these procedures are dangerous, but some beauty doctors won't tell their clients that because they are obsessed with the beauty of fresh dollar notes.

This is where essential oils come into play. Most of these oils have chemical properties that help to rejuvenate the skin and help cell regeneration. Essential oils help oxygen circulate better in the skin, and this oxygen is needed by cells for regeneration. Due to their anti-oxidation quality, some essential oils are known for their ability to eliminate free radicals existing on the skin, which are capable of destroying the molecules of the topmost skin layer.

Some of the most commonly used essential oils for anti-aging procedures include

Clary sage, Frankincense, Palmarosa, Jasmine, Rosemary, Mastic, Violet Leaf, Marjoram, Immortelle, Carrot Seed, Rosewood, Sandalwood, Cistus, Rose Otto, Patchouli, Lavender, Spikenard, Violet leaf, and Ylang ylang.

In using these essential oils to create blends to be used on the face, your considerations should go further than just mixing any of the oils and expecting a result on your face. Some of these oils are best suited for different skin types, and if they used wrongly, it might be hard to get any appreciable results. Before any blend is prepared, a skin test should be carried out to ascertain the skin type so that the best essential oil for the skin can be selected. For example, geranium as an essential is mostly used on dry skin to reduce dryness, remove patches on the skin, and eliminate black lines underneath the eyes. Using geranium on a different type of skin will produce no visible results since the skin has none of the conditions that geranium is known to bring solutions to.

Here are some oil blends that can be used for anti-aging procedures:

The first blend is made by adding three drops of chamomile german, chamomile roman, and lemon. Next, you add two drops of lavender and rosemary oil. Dilute the mixture by adding one tablespoon of carrier oil. Use your finger to stir the blend until the mixture is evenly distributed. Apply gently around the face.

For older skin with deeper and more defined wrinkles, you might need to get a more robust blend to deal with that. To produce that blend you add 3 drops of frankincense oil, 1 drop of rosemary oil, 3 drops of neroli oil, and one drop of immortelle. Add one tablespoon of the carrier oil, mix with your fingers, and apply on the face.

Facial scrub with essential oils
Facial scrubs are very effective when used on the skin to help achieve a smooth and softer feel on the skin. The essential oils used in facial scrubs leave the skin feeling refreshed after such a scrub. You should treat your face to a face scrub at least once every week to get rid of dead skins and allow new ones to come to the surface. Here is a blend you can use:

The first blend used in facial scrub is produced by mixing 3 drops of neroli oil, 3 drops of sandalwood oil, 3 drops of orange oil, and one tablespoon of your selected essential oil. Add three teaspoons of sugar and mix thoroughly with a spoon. Use the mixture to scrub the face for about five minutes, but be careful not to bruise your face since this is a rough mixture. Wash off with mild soap and warm water.

A less harsh scrub for more sensitive skin is made adding 5 drops chamomile oil, 5 drops of lavender oil, 1 tablespoon of oat flour and 3 teaspoons of sugar. Mix the blend thoroughly and add in 1 tablespoon of your selected carrier oil. Apply the scrub on your face using continuous circular motions for about five minutes. Rinse off with warm water and mild soap.

Essential Oils used for Hair Care
Essential oils are also very important in Haircare. A number of them are known to revitalize, smoothen

and add a glossy look when used on the air. This is almost like a secret that only aromatherapists understand. Knowing some of these essential oils and how they can be used will help you deal with stunted hair growth, scanty hair in the middle of the head, and a receding hairline.

A few examples of plant oils which are used for hair care include hemp seed oil which helps to strengthen the scalp and keep it healthy; Moringa, which provides a glossy look to hair texture; Shea Butter, which is best for the damaged scalp; Jojoba, a balancing oil best for scalp treatment. Other oils used for this purpose include camellia seed, avocado oil, sesame oil, borage seed oil, Neem oil, almond oil e.t.c

Best Essential Oils for Different Hair Types

Normal Hair: Geranium, Rosemary, Carrot Seed, Lavender, Cedarwood, and Lemon essential oils.

Dry Hair: Frankincense, Sandalwood, Palmarosa, geranium, and Carrot seed essential oils.

Oily Hair: Cedarwood, Juniper berry, Bergamot, Eucalyptus, Basil linalool, lime, lemon, grapefruit, and Petitgrain essential oils.

The All-Purpose Essential Oil Blend for any hair type
Most times, some essential oils are used in creating blends that will suit a particular hair type, either dry hair, oily hair, aging hair, or sun-damaged hair. This specific blend will be used on all hair kinds to improve hair quality and overall health. You can use

it on your hair if you have no particular condition you want to deal with.

This blend is created using the following 10 drops of Argan oil, 10 drops of Rice bran oil, 1 tablespoon of jojoba oil, and 5 drops of meadowfoam oil. Mix thoroughly with a spoon and apply in a sliding motion over the scalp. You can make a large blend and store it for continuous use.

Essential Oils Blend for Stimulating Hair Growth
For this blend, you will need 10 drops of lavender essential oils, 10 drops of rosemary essential oils, 10 drops of peppermint essential oils, a quarter cup of coconut oils, and another quarter cup of castor oil. First, add castor and coconut oil in a container and mix. Next, add the essential oils. Shake the container until all of the essential oils are evenly distributed in the blend. To apply, massage your scalp using the blend and cover with a shower cap or drag. Wash your head in the morning using organic shampoo. You can make use of this blend at least two times every week for maximum results.

This next blend is created using 3 drops of lavender essential oil, 4 drops of lemon essential oil, 7 drops of rosemary essential oil, 8 drops of coconut carrier oil, and 4 drops of apricot kernel oil. Mix the two carrier oils (the coconut and apricot kernel oil) first and then add in the essential oils. Shake the bottle thoroughly until the essential oils in the blend are evenly distributed. Apply the blend by massaging it directly into the scalp. Keep your hands moving in a circular motion until you feel the oil on your scalp. Allow for an hour before you wash off using shampoo.

Essentials Oils for Hair Cream
For this, you will need 4 tablespoons of shea butter,
1 tablespoon of coconut oil, 1 tablespoon of Olive
Oil, 2 drops of roman chamomile essential oil, 4
drops of rosemary essential oil, 5 drops of
frankincense essential oil and 2 drops of geranium
essential oil. Put the shea butter and coconut oil in a
container and melt in a microwave for some
seconds. Once melted, you can add all of the other
ingredients and mix thoroughly. Allow it to cool, after
which you can use on your hair and store for future
use.

Essential oils for Hair Nourishing Shampoo
This blend is used to add a touch of glossiness and
sheen to the hair. The essential oils used in this
blend are the cypress and helichrysum essential
oils. Helichrysum is known for the healing it provides
on the hair, and cypress helps to reduce the oiliness
of the hair.

To create the blend, you add 4 drops of cypress
essential oil and 4 drops of Helichrysum essential oil
to 6 ounces of bland shampoo. Mix thoroughly and
begin to use.

Essential Oils for Hair Conditioner
This blend helps to soothe the scalp and reduce the
oiliness of the hair. You will need 4 drops of
lavender essential oil, 4 drops of rosemary essential
oil, and 6 ounces of hair conditioner. Add the
essential oils to the conditioner and mix. Make use
of this just after shampooing your hair. Allow it to
remain on the hair for about 2 minutes before
rinsing off.

Chapter Seven: Essential Oils for Home Use

There are hundreds of products in today's market that promise to leave your home smelling calm, homely, and inviting. Sure, lots of them end up getting the job done, while the others, well, do something. But the truth is that none of them can infuse that natural smell into your home, that distinct aroma will forever leave your home more inviting and appeal than ever. This is something most homeowners strive to achieve in their homes. There are several experiments you can carry out with your favorite essential oils. Some of these are also known to prevent the gathering of some rodents and insects. They also come with properties to keep your home looking clean and fresh.

Common Essential Oils for Home Use
Some of the most commonly used essential oils used in-home care include:

Rosemary essential oil, which has antimicrobial properties that can help you halt the activities of microbes on your surfaces, thereby preventing infections. Constant inhalation of this essential oil is known to relieve respiratory tract symptoms such as coughs and catarrh. Rosemary oil can be blended with other essential oils to produce a distinct aroma for your home.

Lemon Essential oil, which can be found as a component of major household cleaning solutions, is among the best oils you can use in-home care. The aroma is fruity and appealing, but that isn't its best quality. Lemon oil also doubles as a disinfectant used in wiping up surfaces. It is crucial for wiping off-odors and the microbes that cause them. Some ways in which lemon oil is used include freshening up the air in the bathroom, cleaning and mopping floors, adding to laundry to make them smell better after washing, cleaning glass windows, and sanitizing sponges.

Eucalyptus Essential Oil is famed for its cleaning power. It is also one of the few essential oils which is known for its undeniable effect on the mind and soul. Eucalyptus is known to help deal with hair infections like dandruff, and when sprinkled in cupboards and wardrobes, it is known to chase out rodents and other forms of pests. Some of the essential components contained in the oil include camphene, pinene, camphor, and citronellol. All of these components have the specific functions that they perform to produce one sizeable powerful output.

Lemongrass Essential Oil has antibacterial qualities that makes it important as a disinfectant. When used, it is known to produce this fresh aroma that projects an image of cleanliness. The aroma is also useful in repelling insects and green snakes. Citral, which is found as a component of lemongrass, has a citrus smell that makes it smell fruity and inviting. Lemongrass oil can be used in the home to improve sleep, repel insects, and freshen the overall atmosphere in the home. The oil can be blended with others such as bergamot, ylang ylang, lime, rosemary, cedarwood, and tea tree oils.

Lime Essential Oil is another oil, which is a major constituent used in the production of cleaning solutions, making a perfect option in germ fighting. This essential oil smells like lemongrass and lemon oil, but it has the most citrusy smell among all of them. The lime oil is also very peculiar among other essential oils for its ability to fight both gram-positive and gram-negative bacteria. Its major chemical component is limonene, which gives lime oil its strong citrus scent. Limonene is also known for its anti-inflammatory and antioxidant qualities. Lime oil helps to alleviate the effect of some respiratory afflictions such as bronchitis. Lime oil can be added to spray solution and sprayed in corners of the houses. There is this clean aroma it produces that gives the home a pleasant and appealing feel.

Parts of the home and essential oils that suit them best

The Bedroom
In considering essential oils for the bedroom, there are two considerations to be made: First, there are essential oils that are used to revitalize the romantic aspect, and there are those blended and used for the sole aim of reducing anxiety and improving sleep. So before you make your decision, you should know what you are going for. You can use any of these blends to satisfy either of the purposes.

For Sleep Enhancement: The blend used for this is made by adding five drops of lavender essential oil, 4 drops of rose essential oil, 5 drops of Geranium essential oil, 2 drops of clary sage, and 6 drops of palmarosa. All of these should be mixed thoroughly and put into a diffuser where it will be released gradually into the atmosphere of the bedroom. If a person suffers from a case of insomnia, you can add sweet orange oil or chamomile oil to the blend to help revive sleep.

Other essential oils that can be used in sleep improvement include sandalwood essential oil, which is very effective in the reduction of anxiety. The oil also produces slight sedative effects when inhaled, reducing alertness and fostering sleepiness. Note that sandalwood oil works differently for people. For some people, the oil is known to increase alertness and repel sleep. Try out the oil at least once to find if it works for you before you begin constant usage.

For Better Romance and Intimacy: Several essential oils are known for their aphrodisiac properties. Some are known to hasten erection in men and arouse women into the sexual mood faster than usual. Some of the include ylang ylang, jasmine, rose, clary sage, neroli, and fennel essential oils.

All of these oils can be used in different ways to produce almost the same effects. Jasmine oil can be blended with everyday massage oils and used on the body of a spouse. Clary sage oil can be inhaled directly from a bottle as an antidepressant for women who have hit menopause. Clary sage essential oil is also known to balance sexual hormones in people with low libido.

The Living Room
For use in the living room, essential oil blends are best used with diffusers to allow the aroma to travel gradually throughout the sitting room space. There are lots of essential oils with a good smell that can be used in the sitting room, so you can select any one of your favorites to use or make a blend with more than one of them. Your sitting room tells so much about your home, and it is probably the place

you spend the most time in, so you might want to take enough time to make a selection of essential oil for it.

Lavender Oil is good for your living room because of the calming and cooling effect its aroma produces when inhaled. The result is a natural one, and it has been described as a mind soothing experience. You can use lavender oil in your diffuser and leave it on throughout the day, or make use of a vaporizer that releases the mixture in vapor form at close intervals, say one hour. You can also add drops of lavender in a spray bottle and spray the cushions before you leave the house or before the arrival of visitors. Raise the cushion foams, and releases drop of your choice oils underneath, then cover and allow the smell to fill the air.

Lime and lemon essential oil are good clean agents for glass windows, to get shiny and sparkly clean. Put 2 drops each of lemon and lime essential oil on a ball of cotton wool and use to rub the surface of the glass window. It will remove stubborn stains and leave the window leaving cleaner than before.

The Bathroom
There are only a few things as good as having a bathroom that isn't only neat but smells nice. Those are probably the best kind of bathrooms. Using essential oils in your bathroom doesn't only help you get rid of germs building up in sinks or walls, it also gives the place a kind of fragrance that makes your bath sessions a little bit more interesting. There is a number of ways in which essential oils can be used in bathrooms. First, you add essential oils into your bathroom diffusers, if you have any or add drops of your select oil in dark corners of the bathroom like

the cupboards that hold the shampoos, soap bars and other toiletries.

Some of the most commonly used essential oils in the bathroom include cinnamon, lemon, citronella, bergamot, thyme, palmarosa and oregano. All of these have aromas that suit the bathroom, and they project this image of cleanliness. You can also create blends from all of these and produce a signature smell for your bathroom. You can be experimental and find out what works for you. Create something that suits your signature, something that visitors coming into your home will never forget. You can try some of these blends in the meantime.

The first is produced using 4 drops of bergamot oil, 8 drops of lemon oil, 7 drops of citronella, 5 drops of oregano, and 2 drops of thyme oil. Mix the blend well enough and apply as desired. You can add drops of the blend into a spray bottle so that.

Another blend can be created using three drops of thyme, 5 drops of cinnamon, and 4 drops of frankincense essential oil. Mix well and apply the blend in your bathroom as desired.

Chapter Eight: Essential Oils for Emotional Wellbeing

Throughout this book, we have studied lots of essential oils and how they can be used in different facets of our lives, from the improvement of physical wellbeing to use in children and use to lighten the overall atmosphere of a home. All of those are important uses that provide even more significant benefits. In this chapter, we will be taking it a bit further and deeper. Before now, we have only considered the physical/tangible benefits of using essential oils. Here we will consider the importance of essential oils in improving emotions, mood, and mental health.

Let's consider some of the most popular and important essential oils used for this purpose, some of which include bergamot, chamomile roman, frankincense, cedarwood, lavender, geranium, clary sage, ylang ylang, petitgrain, and vetiver oils. Some of these can be used alone, or they can be used in combination with each other. Most of them have been in use for centuries, sprinkled around the chambers of kings and royalties to ward off bad spirits and help bring good and peaceful sleep. Some others are also used for the same purpose with amazing results, only that they are expensive. But if you have the resources to afford them, you can go for them. Some of these include neroli, jasmine, hyacinth, carnation, and rose otto essential oils.

Essential Oils for Calmness
There is a number of essential oil blends you can use for this. Some of these should work wonders:

The first blend is produced using 10 drops of bergamot essential oil, 1 drop of juniper essential oil, 1 drop of patchouli essential oil, 4 drops of ylang ylang, and 8 drops of lavender.

First, add the bergamot, juniper, and patchouli essential oils and stir. Allow to rest for about three minutes then add ylang ylang and lavender oils. Lavender is important in this blend because of the sedative effect it produces when inhaled. Before sleep sets in, there will be a brief moment of calmness. The blend can be put into a diffuser so that the room is gradually filled up with the smell. You can add some drops of the blend into your bath water and use it for your night bath just before going to bed.

Another blend that gets the job done is produced using lavender, rose otto, and vanilla essential oils. The vanilla flavor has continuously been associated with pleasantness, sweetness, and beauty. All of these come together to improve mood and alleviate depression. To produce the blend, add 2 drops of vanilla oil, 10 drops of rose otto oil, and 5 drops of lavender. Mix these thoroughly until the blend is uniformly distributed. You can add drops of the blend to a spray bottle quarter-filled with water and shake vigorously. Spray the solution at the back of your neck and under your ribs after bathing at night.

The next blend is produced using 5 drops of vetiver, 10 drops of cedarwood, and 2 drops of ylang ylang oils. You can add the juniper berry essential oil if the person in question is also showing signs of intense restlessness, paranoia, unease, and anxiety. Add the blend to your diffuser and allow the atmosphere to get saturated for the next hour before the individual is allowed to come into the room to sleep.

Finally, you can create a blend using ylang ylang, lavender and roman chamomile essential oils. Chamomile roman has been in use for a long time in fostering calmness in an environment. Ylang ylang as oil has used to help regulate and stabilize the heartbeat, thereby easing anxiety. To create the blend, add 4 drops of lavender, 3 drops of roman chamomile, and 2 drops of ylang ylang essential oils to a bottle. Add drops of the blend to a diffuser or use it in a hot bath.

Essential Oils to help with bereavement
These are essential oils used on people who have just lost someone and who are overwhelmed with sorrow. They help to provide some form of support for people going through the shadow of loss. They are also known to take away sad memories and bring a feeling of hope when inhaled. All of these sound fantastical until you try them out and see the results. In essence, these oils are used to make the mourning process easier. Some of them include melissa, cypress, frankincense, spikenard, cistus, neroli, benzoin, rose otto, mandarin, and patchouli essential oils. Remember that people respond differently to essential oils, so all of these might not trigger the same response from different people.

Some blends that can be used for bereavement include using 3 drops of rose oil, 3 drops of Helichrysum oil, 3 drops of cypress, and 5 drops of frankincense.

Another blend can be made by adding 4 drops of Neroli oil, 4 drops of rose oil, and 5 drops of sandalwood oil.

After mixing all of these thoroughly to get your desired blend, add drops of the blend into a diffuser while following all instructions given by the manufacturer. Allow the blend to remain in the diffuser overnight until the whole room is filled with the aroma.

Essential Oils for Stress Control
Essential oils are perfect for relieving stress at the end of a hectic day or after going through some major trauma. They can be used in a bath, for massage, or inhaled from diffusers. Some of the major oils used for this purpose include coriander essential oil, patchouli essential oil, lavender, tea tree, vanilla, and clary sage essential oils.

The first blend used for this can be made using 4 drops of bergamot oil, 2 drops of patchouli, 8 drops of lavender oil, 3 drops of coriander, and 1 tablespoon of carrier oil. Bergamot and coriander oil is known to relieve stress levels and foster inspiration. Mix thoroughly and store for continuous use. You can use it for massages or add to your bathwater.

A blend made with lemon, lime, frankincense, and neroli essential oils is good as it is used to calm an agitated, confused, or confused spirit. You can create the blend by adding 5 drops of frankincense, 3 drops of neroli, and 5 drops of lemon and lime essential oils. This blend can be used with a carrier oil to massage the lower abdomen, the temple, and the back of the neck. It can also be dropped into warm water and used for bath.

Grapefruit essential oil is known for its uplifting qualities and for the surge of mental boost it provides. Its aroma helps people deal with negative and fearful thoughts. It is even enhanced when it is used as a blend alongside other essential oils like juniper berry and rosemary. The blend is created by adding three drops of all and mixing thoroughly. The blend can be used in a diffuser or in a hot bath.

Essential Oils for Depression
The essential oils majorly used in dealing with depression include lavender, jasmine, vanilla, sandalwood, ylang ylang, grapefruit, ginger, and bergamot essential oils. For instance, ginger oil is known to contain chemical compounds with antidepressant qualities. Research has shown that inhaling ginger oil has a way of dealing with stress-induced depression. Ginger oil activates the activities of the serotonergic system, which coordinates the brain transmission process, thereby leading to the release of stress-control hormones. Bergamot essential is known for its uplifting quality. The oil reduced mental complications that may result from intense depression in an individual.

These essential oils can be used as blends or alone. Choosing to inhale them straight from the bottle or to allow them gradually saturate the atmosphere depends totally on your decision. But you can make a choice based on what works best for you. For some users, inhaling the aroma directly from the bottle always produces a stronger reaction than when they are placed in diffusers and allowed to saturate the atmosphere. For others, the reverse is the case. You can use other methods like adding drops of your select oil to cotton wool and inhaling at intervals or adding some drops to your bathwater. Some blends that can be used for depression include:

The first one is made by adding 5 drops of bergamot essential oil, 4 drops of helichrysum essential oil and 5 drops of ylang ylang essential oil, in that order. You can add the blend to your diffuser or mix with distilled water in a spray bottle and spray the mixture around the corners of the room.

Another blend can be made using 7 drops of roman chamomile essential oil, 5 drops of sandalwood essential oil and 4 drops of ginger oil. Whenever ginger oil comes in contact with roman chamomile essential oil, they produce this aroma that is at once appealing and stress relieving. Note that this blend doesn't always produce the same effect when used on different people. For some people, it helps provide clarity and freedom from a depressive mood; for others, it leaves them without any significant change. First, try the combination by using small quantities of the essential oils and noting your reaction to the blend. If it is a positive one, then you can go ahead and create the blend in larger quantities for continuous usage.

The final blend to be discussed is a massage blend. You can do this by adding 6 drops of bergamot essential oil and 2 drops each of grapefruit and sandalwood oil. Mix thoroughly until the essential oils are evenly distributed in the blend. Take a few drops of the blend and rub all over your palms. Massage the back of your neck, the base of your skull, and your shoulders. You can get somebody to help you out with the massage you that you get the right spots massaged well enough.

Conclusion

We have been blessed by nature, and one way in which this blessing manifests itself is in the availability of essential oils that serve hundreds of purposes, most of which have been revealed to you in this book. From all the procedures and processes outlined in this book, it is easy to understand and see that you don't need to be a professional before you can make use of the beauty that lies in essential oils. You can tap into this resource anytime and benefit from it. Start using the most common oils in your house and notice the positive change of mood before you start going for other values. Instead of going for artificial air fresheners, you can make use of nature's aroma and leave your home smelling more natural than normal.

As you use the oils, try to understand them better. With time you can add more of them to your collection and broaden your scope of usage. Use them for a variety of purposes like some of the ones that have been listed here in the book. Occasionally, you may want to return to this book as a reminder or a manual to help you remember some of the procedures.

Don't hesitate to try out blends when you feel inspired. All of the blends that are listed in this book came to people during moments of inspiration, and the same can happen to you, too, so don't restrict yourself. Don't forget to take the notes and grades of the oils into consideration when creating blends. Both of these will help you develop better blends with a more uniform aroma.

In ending, remember to take caution when purchasing your oils. There are lots of adulterated forms of your favorite essential oils flooding the market. Some of these are capable of leaving you with adverse negative effects, so you'd need to be careful. Don't neglect the advice provided in chapter one of this book on purchasing and storing your oils. Once you come across a reputable and trustworthy seller, you stick to them. Making use of quality essential oils only makes the aromatherapy experience sweeter and more interesting.